Create Your Own Kidney Diet Plan

Build A Meal Pattern For Stage 3 or 4 Kidney Disease

Mathea Ford, RD/LD

Introduction and Disclaimer

I wrote this book with you in mind: the person with kidney problems who does not know where to start or can't seem to get the answers that you need from other sources. I am writing this book to help you manage your kidney disease and make it easier to live with by giving you answers [in general] to questions that you have.

This book will tell you what to eat and how to choose the right foods for your meals. I will go in depth about how to eat and how to plan what you should have for the day.

Who am I? I am a registered dietitian in the USA who has been working with kidney patients for my entire 15 + years of experience. I have a website that provides renal diet meal plans for all stages of kidney disease – learn more at http://www.renaldiethq.com/predialysis-book/

My meal plans are very popular, and I felt that I needed to give back and help you travel down the road with a little more information than you had before. Forgive me if I get a little technical, I am going to do my best to get the information to you that you need.

My goals are simple – to give some answers and to create an understanding of what is typical. It will not necessarily be what happens in your case, as everyone is an individual. I may simplify things in an effort to write them so that I feel you can learn the most from the information. This may mean that I don't say the exact things that your doctor would say. If you don't understand, please ask your doctor.

I want you to understand, I am not a medical doctor and I do not know your particular condition. Information in this book is current as of publication, but may or may not have changed. This book is not meant to substitute for medical treatment for you, your friends, or your family members. You should not base treatment decisions solely on what is contained in this book. Develop your treatment plan with your doctors, nurses and the other medical professionals on your team. I recommend that you double-check any information with your medical team to verify if it applies to you.

In other words, I am not responsible for your medical care. I am providing this book for information and entertainment purposes, not medical diagnoses. Please consult with your doctor about any questions that you have about your particular case.

Table Of Contents

You get FREE nutritional information on regular food items – from Alcohol to Vegetables and on Fast Food items. It is hard to put them in a book, so I have a link for you to go and download them from. They are sorted by sodium, potassium and phosphorus amounts for the standard food items. The fast food items do not have potassium and phosphorus amounts, so they are sorted alphabetically. You also get the excel spreadsheet that I use in the book as we work through the meal plan – you will need that to work through the examples in the book. Just enter your email address and once you confirm, they will come to you in your inbox.

The reason why I have you give me an email is that if I find a problem with the worksheets, I can send you an updated version. You will also get a notification when I publish additional books on renal diet topics. At any time, you can unsubscribe from the list and you will get no further emails from me.

http://www.renaldiethq.com/predialysis-book/files-for-create-your-own-kidney-diet-book/

For reference, I used the K/DOQI Nutrition In Chronic Renal Failure Guidelines which are the guidelines for doctors and dietitians to use to provide evidence based practice and nutritional care.

American Journal of Kidney Diseases, Vol 35, No 6, Suppl 2 (June), 2000

What is Kidney Disease?

Approximately 23 Million US Adults have Chronic Kidney Disease. That is an average of 11% of the population, a little over one in 10 people, but it is estimated that half of them do not even know it! Kidney disease is treatable, but it can be harmful and painful as well. You do not have to suffer – but you have to know how to get more help. In this book, I use the word renal and kidney somewhat interchangeably. If I say kidney disease in one paragraph and renal disease in the next, it is the same condition.

I want you to know that you can stop or slow down the progression of this disease with a proper diet and some medications from your doctor for the related conditions. This book is about how to develop a proper diet.

Most people who have kidney disease develop the damage over time as a result of either diabetes or high blood pressure. Diabetes is a major cause of kidney failure, and uncontrolled diabetes wreaks havoc on the small capillaries in your kidneys. Uncontrolled high blood pressure does the same thing to the small blood vessels inside your kidneys that filter blood and waste from your body. The progression of the disease is difficult to understand because it doesn't hurt – meaning you don't have pain at that time that your kidneys are being damaged. But the damage is being done day by day when you have diabetes or high blood pressure every time that you don't manage to get them under control.

What Do Diabetes and High Blood Pressure Have To Do With Kidney Disease?

Main risks that lead to the development of kidney disease are high blood pressure, obesity and diabetes mellitus. When kidney disease is not detected early, you lose the ability to delay the onset of further damage and possibly continue to cause additional damage when it could have easily been prevented.

Think of your risk factors for developing kidney disease as either modifiable or non-modifiable. Risk factors that are modifiable (or can be changed) are blood pressure, blood sugar, blood cholesterol, smoking, alcohol use, dietary changes, medication misuse, and obesity. Risk factors that are not modifiable are your age, gender, race, and genetics. As you age, you have a natural decline in kidney function that is not necessarily harmful nor always in need of treatment. When you finally realize you have kidney disease, it may be fairly far along. However, if you are able to have your blood tested early – especially if you have some risk factors – you stand a much better chance of lower risk of hospitalization and advancing disease than those who find out too late. Early education and actions to intervene are important to slow the progression of chronic kidney disease.

Basically, over 40% of people who develop kidney disease have diabetes, and kidney disease is an important risk factor for heart disease. The diseases are intertwined and affect each other. If you have uncontrolled diabetes, you are putting yourself at risk of developing kidney disease sooner rather than later. You also have a more difficult (although not impossible) time of managing it.

As a diabetic, you need to control your diabetes first and foremost. When your diabetes is not well controlled, meaning your hemoglobin A1c is above 7.5%, you have damage to your kidneys. Suffice it to say that your red blood cells (the hemoglobin in hemoglobin A1c) become very large when they have glucose attached to them. That is what your A1c is measuring – the amount of glucose attached to red blood cells. The higher your blood glucose level, the more glucose (sugar) attaches to your red blood cells and makes them large. These as well as the high amounts of sugar in your blood lead to damage in your kidneys.

For high blood pressure, the damage happens over time and you probably don't even notice it. You have extra pressure on the small blood vessels in your kidneys (known as nephrons and capillaries), which cause them to become damaged. You don't feel this damage. But over time, less and less of your kidneys are working which is why you have impairment.

Your doctor may tell you that you have 20% function or 50% function, and what they mean is that is the amount of your kidneys that don't have damaged nephrons and capillaries. The good news is that you really don't usually need dialysis until you reach 10% or less function.

Persons with kidney disease should maintain a blood pressure reading of 130/90 or lower – preferably in the 120/80 range. You should work with your doctor or nephrologist (kidney disease specialist) to get the blood pressure down to an acceptable level to decrease the additional damage that is being done when it is too high.

Other Causes of Kidney Disease

Some people are born with a condition called polycystic kidney disease (PKD). This means that their kidneys develop cysts which slowly replace normally functioning kidneys. This leads to kidney failure over time. If you are concerned that you have PKD, because a family member has it, you should discuss it with your family doctor.

Other things, such as medication or autoimmune diseases can affect your kidneys. You should avoid certain medications – like NSAID's (Ibuprofen for one) when you have kidney disease.

One chronic disease that can affect many parts of your body but your kidneys as well is Lupus. Lupus is a chronic inflammation and this can cause damage to the small blood cells in the kidneys. If you have lupus, be sure to have your kidneys checked regularly for functioning.

Finally, you could have a few other reasons that I will not mention. But, you are reading this book because you need a kidney diet for someone who has stages 3-5 kidney disease. You need to do a few things to help them out.

First, Determine Your Stage of Kidney Disease

First, let me tell you about the different stages of kidney disease. The definition of chronic kidney disease is decreased function of the kidney or kidney damage that lasts 3 months or longer. Most stages of kidney disease are rated based on Glomerular Filtration Rate (GFR) or estimated GFR (eGFR). Normal kidney function is an eGFR of 90 or above. Doctors may also test for presence of protein in the urine to validate the eGFR or get a better picture of the amount of damage and risk for progression to higher stages of kidney disease.

How do they calculate eGFR? Doctors and labs can estimate the GFR based on the amount of creatinine in your blood stream. The calculation is made based on the milligrams of creatinine in one deciliter of blood (mg/dL). They then use the patient's information about their age, sex and race to estimate the GFR. A regular GFR rate requires an injection of a substance and a collection of 24 hours worth of urine to determine. I think you will agree that the eGFR is a good way to start.

In this section, I am just going to explain the kidney disease stages and how to understand how serious it is.

Stage 1 Kidney Disease

Kidney damage with an eGFR ≥ 90 ml/min is considered stage 1 kidney disease. It is important to note that most people do not even realize they have kidney disease at this stage. You may not have symptoms at this point, nor do you have to change a lot about your diet and activity.

Stage 2 Kidney Disease

Kidney damage with an eGFR of 60-89 ml/min is considered stage 2 kidney disease. You have mild kidney disease, but note that if you have protein in your urine (trace, 1+ or 2+) you need to be assertive and discuss with your doctor how to slow down the process of moving to stage 3 kidney disease.

Stage 3 Kidney Disease

An eGFR of 30-59 ml/min is considered stage 3 kidney disease, with or without known damage. You have moderate to severe kidney disease, and you probably have protein in your urine. At this stage, it is recommended that when your GFR gets close to 30 mL/min that you are referred to a nephrologist (specialist in kidney disease) for co-management with your personal physician.

Stage 4 Kidney Disease

When you have an eGFR of 15-29 ml/min it is considered stage 4 kidney disease. You can continue to make the important dietary and medical changes that your doctor recommends to reduce the rate of the progression to dialysis. You are on the doorstep of dialysis and should realize that you need to take drastic action if you have not done so up to now.

Stage 5 Kidney Disease

Stage 5 kidney disease is when your eGFR falls below 15 ml/min. You are at about 10% of your kidneys capacity still functional. You are likely to be preparing for dialysis at this time. It is not the end of the world if you are on dialysis, and as a matter of fact, many people who have been sick for so long can find dialysis makes them feel better because the waste product is being removed from their blood on a regular basis.

Some people think that Stage 5 kidney disease is also dialysis, but dialysis is a step beyond Stage 5. You have to be diagnosed as having end stage renal disease. This means that your kidneys no longer function enough to sustain life. You need assistance. You have a few options, and you need to be as healthy as possible prior to reaching this stage.

Now, How Do I Manage My Diet?

If you want to manage your diet ins stages 1-2, it is recommended to control your related conditions – whether it be high blood pressure or diabetes. It is also recommended to follow the DASH diet (Dietary Approaches To Stopping Hypertension). Stages 3 – 5 are really where you start to limit certain nutrients for your condition. So, if you are in stages 1 or 2 of kidney failure, please work hard on lowering your blood pressure or keeping your blood sugars under control.

I am going to explain to you about how to control the salt, protein, potassium, and phosphorus in your diet because these are the nutrients that are a problem for you and will cause further kidney damage. I am also going to give you specifics on what foods have high amounts of potassium, salt and phosphorus so you can use them sparingly (*in the download that you get for free with this book*).

So, I will help you get started and help you have many more choices than you ever thought you could. While the diet is a little bit complicated, I want you to do as much as you can to have control over your health and changing your diet will help with this. I hope that you will find it easy enough to make the changes I talk about. I am even going to go into eating out!

Reading Nutritional Labels

When you first start planning your meals, you will come across something that looks like this (in the USA). It tells you a lot of information about the product and serving sizes. I am going to dissect this food label for you and review the information that you will need to understand and pay attention to when you are reading them in the stores and in your homes..

Nutrition Facts

Serving Size 1 cup (228g)
Servings per Container 2

Amount Per Serving

Calories 280	Calories from Fat 120

	% Daily Value*
Total Fat 13g	20%
Saturated Fat 5g	25%
Trans Fat 2g	
Cholesterol 2mg	10%
Sodium 660mg	28%
Total Carbohydrate 31g	10%
Dietary Fiber 3g	0%
Sugars 5g	
Protein 5g	

Vitamin A 4%	•	Vitamin C 2%
Calcium 15%	•	Iron 4%

Percent Daily Values are based on a 2,000-calorie diet. Your daily values may be higher or lower depending on your calorie needs.

	Calories:	2,000	2,500
Total Fat	Less than	65g	80g
Sat Fat	Less than	20g	25g
Cholesterol	Less than	300mg	300mg
Sodium	Less than	2,400mg	2,400mg
Total Carbohydrate		300g	375g
Fiber		25g	30g

Calories per gram:

Fat 9 • Carbohydrate 4 • Protein 4

First of all, it is required on most all foods, except for things like fresh fruit and other fresh produce (which are items that you need to understand the amount of potassium and phosphorus contained in a serving) These items may have a general guideline for the food item located near the product for you to look at.

Lets get started at the top of the label –

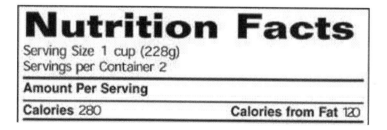

Nutrition Facts

Serving Size 1 cup (228g)
Servings per Container 2

Amount Per Serving

Calories 280	Calories from Fat 120

This label is telling us that in one cup of this product, we will have 280 calories. Important to also note – the package contains 2 servings. SO if we eat the entire package, we need to realize that we will need to double all the numbers in the nutrition label to get an accurate amount of food and calories eaten.

You may not have realized that you still need to exercise, quit smoking and keep reading about your condition. Do as much as possible to stay healthy, including saying no to a second portion if you have some weight to lose.

Next up –

Amount Per Serving	
Calories 280	Calories from Fat 120
	% Daily Value*
Total Fat 13g	20%
Saturated Fat 5g	25%
Trans Fat 2g	
Cholesterol 2mg	10%

Either way, you will see that we have fat – Both saturated and trans-fat, in our label. Can't really escape it. So in this 1 cup serving, you have 280 calories and 13 grams of fat. As a person on a renal diet, that may be ok. You are trying to reduce the amount of protein in your diet, and if you are a diabetic, you might have to manage your carbohydrate as well. But you should try to eat lower fat as well. Heart disease is another risk you face with kidney disease. So, this one is probably high, especially if you eat the whole package since you will need to double the amounts.

Look at the daily value. That amount is based on the recommended amount for a person on a 2000 calorie diet. In this case, it's 20% of the daily value (the total amount they recommend you eat is 65 gm of fat). That may be high or low, depending on how many calories you need. In this case, I don't believe the daily value adds a lot to your understanding for this nutrient.

For salt the daily value is very relevant!

Either way, you want to limit the amount of these items in your diet.

But the most important nutrients that you need to consider how much and how many of are the protein, carbohydrate, and sodium.

Sodium 660mg		28%
Total Carbohydrate 31g		10%
Dietary Fiber 3g		0%
Sugars 5g		
Protein 5g		
Vitamin A 4%	•	Vitamin C 2%
Calcium 15%	•	Iron 4%

Percent Daily Values are based on a 2,000-calorie diet. Your daily values may be higher or lower depending on your calorie needs.

Here you can see the sodium in this product is WAYYY too high for someone in need of a renal or kidney diet. If the 660 mg per serving did not provide enough evidence, you can see the daily value. The daily value represents the percentage of the recommended 2,400 mg of sodium for any healthy person. So, even though you should probably eat a lower amount than that, you can consider anything over 20-23% of the daily value to be too high for you to eat. Sodium daily value number is a quick and easy way to see how this food will work in a renal or heart diet – you should aim for less than 20% of the daily value in a food.

In this case, if it was something you really wanted, I might recommend that you cut the serving in half. (So you would eat 1/4th of the package).

Looking further down the label, you can see the amount of protein and carbohydrate as well as dietary fiber. You should try to consume a high amount of fiber daily – in the range of 25 gm of fiber per day. This helps to keep you regular and keeps you feeling full.

The amount of protein in this product is reasonable at 5 gm per serving, depending on the amount of protein that you need per day. I will show you how to calculate that in the next chapter.

The nutrients listed at the bottom of the label such as iron, calcium, and Vitamin C are important to know, but in this case don't add a lot of value to your understanding of the label.

The rest of the label deals with the Daily Value recommendations. This may not be on all labels depending on how much room is available to the manufacturer.

	Calories:	2,000	2,500
Total Fat	Less than	65g	80g
Sat Fat	Less than	20g	25g
Cholesterol	Less than	300mg	300mg
Sodium	Less than	2,400mg	2,400mg
Total Carbohydrate		300g	375g
Fiber		25g	30g
Calories per gram:			
Fat 9 •	Carbohydrate 4	•	Protein 4

At first this appears to be confusing (if you ask me). This is recommended dietary intakes for certain nutrients based on a 2000 or 2500 calorie diet.

It says less than 65 gm of total fat, for example. This is an upper limit. By an upper limit I mean that you should eat no more than this amount. For fiber, it's a recommended amount to reach. This is a high level of fiber, and most Americans do not get this amount.

This is why I feel that the sodium daily value is a very easy way to evaluate whether something is too high in sodium. If you have something that is 10% of your daily value, it's probably ok. But you have to eat more items that are low in sodium and very few that are over 200 mg of sodium.

So, you should always read your labels and understand what you are eating. Now that you have kidney disease, you need to watch what you eat closely and try to stay within your limits.

What Are The Calorie Levels and Limits For My Diet?

You need to determine the amount of each type of nutrient that you can eat. The nutrients that you are concerned with are calories, carbohydrate, protein, sodium (salt), potassium and phosphorus. Some of those nutrients will be prescribed by your doctor and others you can calculate on your own.

USE WORKSHEET LABELED "Calculate Calories" for this section

Calorie Needs:

You can calculate your calorie needs using an equation as dietitians do.

English BMR Formula

Women: BMR = 655 + (4.35 x weight in pounds) + (4.7 x height in inches) - (4.7 x age in years)

Men: BMR = 66 + (6.23 x weight in pounds) + (12.7 x height in inches) - (6.8 x age in year)

Metric BMR Formula

Women: BMR = 655 + (9.6 x weight in kilos) + (1.8 x height in cm) - (4.7 x age in years)

Men: BMR = 66 + (13.7 x weight in kilos) + (5 x height in cm) - (6.8 x age in years)

I got this table from the following website:

http://www.bmi-calculator.net/bmr-calculator/bmr-formula.php

So, you can calculate how many calories you need from this formula. The only issue is if you are overweight. You need to know your healthy body weight. Use the following tables to determine your healthy body weight.

For women and men, you should add 1 inch to your height to be on the right line. Now, it does refer to different size frames for men and women. I think if you are "large boned" you know it. But for most people, they are in the medium frame range. So I would recommend using the middle numbers.

If you are overweight according to the chart, you should do the following:

Take your current weight, subtract your ideal weight (weight from chart) and take that number times .25. Then you add the number you came up with to your ideal body weight number. The number you end up with should be added to your ideal weight. This accounts for the energy that your additional weight needs to function. It's a low number because most of your extra weight is usually fat.

Step 1: Use the provided spreadsheet and enter your numbers to determine your adjusted body weight if needed.

WOMEN				MEN			
Height		**Frame Size**		**Height**		**Frame Size**	
Ft. In.	**Small**	**Med.**	**Large**	**Ft. In.**	**Small**	**Med.**	**Large**
4'10"	102-111	109-121	118-131	5'2"	128-134	131-141	138-150
4'11"	103-113	111-123	120-134	5'3"	130-136	133-143	140-153
5'0"	104-115	113-126	122-137	5'4"	132-138	135-145	142-156
5'1"	106-118	115-129	125-140	5'5"	134-140	137-148	144-160
5'2"	108-121	118-132	128-143	5'6"	136-142	139-151	146-164
5'3"	111-124	121-135	131-147	5'7"	138-145	142-154	149-168
5'4"	114-127	124-138	134-151	5'8"	140-148	145-157	152-172
5'5"	117-130	127-141	137-155	5'9"	142-151	156-160	155-176
5'6"	120-133	130-144	140-159	5'10"	144-154	151-163	158-180
5'7"	123-136	133-144	143-163	5'11"	146-157	154-166	161-184
5'8"	126-139	136-150	146-167	6'0"	149-160	157-170	164-188
5'9"	129-142	139-153	149-170	6'1"	152-164	160-174	168-192
5'10"	132-145	142-156	152-173	6'2"	155-168	165-178	172-197
5'11"	135-148	145-159	155-176	6'3"	158-172	167-182	176-202
6'0"	138-151	148-162	158-176	6'4"	162-176	171-187	181-207

Step 2. At this point, you can **enter your numbers into the spreadsheet** in the blue sections labeled – weight in pounds, height in inches, age in years. Enter your adjusted body weight you just calculated if you are overweight.

So, to complete an example for you for a man and a woman:

Woman: Age 60, 5' 3" tall (including 1 inch for height chart), weight 220 pounds. Her ideal weight is: 128 pounds. (I took the middle of the medium range).

So – 220 pounds – 128 pounds = 92 pounds x .25 = 23 pounds. Add that amount to ideal weight: 128 + 23= 151 pounds to use in calculations – including information about how much protein to eat.

Man: Age 60, 6'2" tall (including 1 inch height for the height chart), weight 250 pounds. His ideal weight is: 172 pounds. (I took the middle of the medium range).

So – 250 pounds – 172 pounds = 78 pounds x .25 = 19.5 pounds. Add that amount to ideal weight: 172 pounds + 19.5 pounds = 192 pounds (rounded up) to use in calculations for calories and protein amounts.

Now, let's calculate their calorie needs so we can figure out how much to feed them, using equation from box above. I will round up or down the decimal points in case you are wondering where they are going.

Woman: 655+ (4.35 x 151 pounds) + (4.7 x 63 inches) – (4.7 x 60 years old) =

655 + 657 + 296 – 282 = 1326 calories for the day

Man: 66 + (6.23 x 192 pounds) + (12.7 x 74 inches) – (6.8 x 60 years old) =

66 + 1196 + 940 – 408 = 1794 calories for the day

(I hope this helps you be able to figure your own calorie needs)

[The spreadsheet provides both men and women numbers – you should use the one that you need based on the sex of the person that you are calculating this for]

Remember, these calculations are not exact but are a good number for you to use. Based on your activity level and amount of muscle weight, you could need a higher number of calories.

Step 3. The spreadsheet automatically gives you the numbers for different activity levels based on your calculated needs. The basic calorie number is the number that you need to lay in bed and rest all day. So you need to multiply the number by 1.1 – 1.5 depending on your activity level. This will be a judgment call on your part, but you should add some for activity. If you find you are losing weight, you will want to add calories to make sure you are at the right amount of calories you need to maintain your weight.

My sample man and woman are walking 30 minutes 3 days a week and still work full time jobs. So I am going to give them an activity factor of 1.2.

Final calorie levels:

Woman: 1326 x 1.2 = 1591 calories

Man: 1794 x 1.2 = 2153 calories for the day.

[The spreadsheet gives you numbers for calories needed based on activity level and if you need to lose weight. Use your judgment about which number is best for you]

Protein Needs

Now that you know how many calories you need, it's easy to figure out the amount of protein you should eat as well.

You have already done the hard work!

Step 4. The spreadsheet will calculate this for you automatically. Or you can do it by just taking your (adjusted) weight in pounds, divide by 2.2 to get your weight in kilograms, and multiply by 0.8.

Woman: 151 pounds / 2.2 = 68.6 kilograms, 68.6 kg x 0.8 = 55 gm protein per day.

Male: 192 pounds / 2.2 = 87.2 kilograms, 87.2 kg x 0.8 = 70 gm of protein per day.

This is a recommended maximum level. You should not exceed this amount of protein in a day. Now, fruits, vegetables and grains have protein in them, and if you are exceeding your protein allowance it should only be with protein from non-animal sources.

But we will get further into how much protein is in each type of food later in this book.

Sodium Limitations

All persons with kidney disease should limit themselves to 2000 mg of sodium per day or less. That will be a difficult number to achieve, and you will need to cook a lot more food at home to make that happen. If your doctor wants you to eat a lower number for sodium, you should follow his/her directions.

Sodium is universal, it is not just salt that you add to food. Sodium is found in many products, especially processed foods. Since you know how to read a label and find sodium on the label, you will need to understand your limits and how you can reduce the amount of sodium that you eat.

You may have heard that sea salt and kosher salt are better for you. The truth is that they all contain sodium. Table salt is a very fine crystal that easily mixes into foods and has a strong taste. Sea salt is made by evaporating sea water, and the mineral crystals of salt that are left are larger than regular table salt. Kosher salt is also a very rough and larger crystal of salt. Kosher salt does tend to have a lower amount of sodium per same measure, but you may find yourself using more because of the taste that you are used to.

It's best to eliminate all additional salt from your diet to help reduce your blood pressure and save your kidneys. Read your labels on all salt products to determine how much you can use.

Potassium Limitations

Limiting your potassium is important to learning to live with kidney disease. Early on in kidney disease, your kidneys may have no problem dealing with any amount of potassium that you throw at them. But as you advance in kidney disease, you will need to lower the amounts of potassium you eat.

Potassium is a mineral that controls nerve and muscle function. One very important muscle — the heart — beats at a normal rhythm because of potassium. In addition, potassium is necessary for maintaining fluid and electrolyte balance and pH level.

In order for potassium to perform these functions, blood levels must be kept between 3.5 and 5.5 mEq/L. The kidneys help keep potassium at a normal level. Potassium levels that are too high or too low can be dangerous.

Your doctor will do blood tests and tell you if you need to lower the amount of potassium in your diet or not. You can do your part by being aware of what foods you eat that contain potassium and limiting them if you need to. It is mainly people with stage 5 kidney disease and on dialysis that need to control their potassium.

Phosphorus Limitations

The kidneys help regulate the level of phosphorus in your blood. If your kidney function is impaired, eventually you will likely have elevated phosphorus levels (hyperphosphatemia). In turn, the elevated phosphorus decreases the level of calcium in your blood, which can lead to bone disease.

Often, 800 to 1,000 milligrams (mg) of phosphorus a day is the limit for someone who has kidney disease in a later stage, like stage 4 or 5. Most healthy adults may eat double this amount. You should discuss with your doctor what amount of phosphorus you should have, and try to manage it by lowering the high phosphorus foods that you may be eating, like dark colas.

Nearly every food contains some phosphorus, so you can't eliminate all phosphorus from your diet. Generally foods high in protein (some meats, dairy products, beans, legumes, nuts and seeds) are higher in phosphorus. Therefore, unless you're receiving kidney dialysis, you'll be asked to eat smaller quantities of them. Whole grains also are higher in phosphorus, so choose refined ones.

How Do I Eat A Lower Salt Diet?

Sodium is found in many preserved and processed foods. The products use salt to help the food stay fresh or preserved for longer. **Any sort of canned product is likely to have more salt** in it than a fresh or frozen product of the same type.

Let's start with talking about how much sodium or salt that you should eat. Most people think of salt and sodium interchangeably but they are actually two different things. Salt is actually a combination of two minerals – sodium and chloride. But I want to concentrate on the sodium. Reading labels is vital to your understanding of just how much sodium you are eating every day. In an earlier section, I discussed how to read labels and what the daily values mean. As a person with a need for a renal diet, you need to stick to about 2,000 mg of sodium per day.

Sodium is found in many foods, so you are not going to ever totally eliminate it from your diet. But it's important to eat the right foods that are not going to have more sodium than you need. Most sodium is found in preserved foods, such as pickles and smoked or canned meats.

Canned vegetables are also a source of high amounts of sodium because of the way they process the vegetables. The difference between fresh corn (1 mg/ear) and canned corn (384 mg/cup) are astounding. And soups are almost your entire day's allowance in one can!

Commercially prepared condiments, like ketchup and mustard or barbeque sauce can be sources of large amounts of sodium. You may want to look for the low sodium versions and possibly start making some of them at home. Cheese is another culprit, and you should watch the amount on the label to see how much sodium each slice contains. You can buy low sodium cheese, and cheddar cheese tends to be lower in sodium than American cheese – but read your labels.

On labels, manufacturers can use certain language to indicate to you that foods are lower in sodium and make you aware of a healthier choice.

- Sodium Free – Less than 5 mg of sodium per serving
- Very Low Sodium – 35 mg of sodium or less per serving
- Low Sodium – 140 mg of sodium or less per serving
- Reduced or Lower Sodium – At least 25% less sodium than the reference food. For example, lower sodium potato chips would have 25% less sodium than regular potato chips.

So, you should be on the lookout for these labels to help you identify healthier foods for you to eat. Compare the lower sodium canned vegetables to their counterparts in the frozen food section, and you will see a big difference.

Getting the salt out of your diet will be difficult in many ways. Our sense of taste has led us to believe that salt is flavor. When it is really just one of many flavors. You will need to try out different seasonings and give it some time to not feel like you are completely missing all flavor in foods.

Ways that you can reduce the sodium in foods that you eat are:

- Eat foods in the least processed state possible. Buy fresh fruits and vegetables if available.
- Frozen vegetables and fruits are low in sodium as well and let you have a variety of options throughout the year
- Use olive oil when cooking to eliminate the salt that is in butter and margarine
- Read your food labels to see how much salt is contained in a serving and don't eat those with more than 20% of your daily value
- Season foods with herbs and spices that do not contain salt. Try ethnic seasoning blends and flavors
- Don't use salt substitutes that claim to be "no salt" or "Nu salt" – if they are white in color they are likely potassium chloride which is just as bad for you (as a kidney patient) as salt
- Ask your doctor about the sodium content of medications that you take
- Adjust your recipes to use less salt than called for

- ➢ Remove the salt shaker from your table and replace it with a seasoning blend
- ➢ Plan your meals ahead of time so you can make sure and have plenty of flavor and variety
- ➢ Use lime or lemon juice to flavor rice and vegetables
- ➢ Make some of your own condiments or buy the lower sodium versions
- ➢ Don't add salt when cooking pasta, rice, vegetables or hot cereals.
- ➢ If you use canned vegetables, pour out the water from the can and rinse the vegetables before cooking to reduce the sodium amount by 60% or more

Condiments can be a big source of sodium. Some are obvious, like onion salt and garlic salt. Use the jar of garlic that is already chopped in the store to flavor dishes. Bouillon cubes and chicken or beef broth are high in sodium, buy the lower sodium versions or make the broth yourself. Baking soda contains a lot of sodium, as does ketchup, barbeque sauce, steak sauce, mustard, soy sauce, Worcestershire sauce, salad dressings, pickles, relish and chili sauces. Do without or make your own if you cannot find a lower sodium version.

Some of my favorite spices to use are cumin, basil, oregano, Italian seasoning, rosemary, and vinegar or lemon juice for vegetables. You can also use lemon juice and a bit of oil on your salad instead of salad dressing.

How Do I Make A Good Meal?

You can make a great meal without salt and that fits your needs for a renal

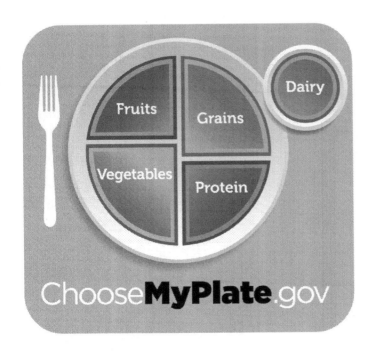

diet. One of the best ways to frame your meal is this:

Think of your plate like this picture. This is the new My Plate educational training by the US Dept of Agriculture. But it's a great example for you too!

You should eat only about ¼ of your plate with protein type foods – so your meats or poultry. That's about 3 ounces. You should fill the rest of your plate with vegetables and fruits that are high in fiber and fit a renal diet – I will give you a list later in the book. And you should eat a small amount of grain or pasta with your meals – it is recommended that you do not eat whole grain pastas if you need lower potassium. And the dairy – only 1 meal per day. Other wise drink a beverage that is recommended like water and only drink the amount that your fluid restriction (if you have one) allows.

Stop thinking about dessert as a sweet thing and realize that you need to balance your diet and eat those types of foods sparingly. You can make the fruit a dessert most of the time, and every now and then splurge on a "sweet". Or you can just skip dessert and be ok.

Lets talk a little bit about how you should eat. If you are overweight, you will need to lose some weight to get to a healthier level. Losing even 10% of your weight will improve your blood pressure and diabetes if you have them. Eating a plate like I described above will lend itself to losing weight because the majority of the food on that plate will be low calorie items, and you will eat more fiber.

The vegetables and fruit are high in fiber and relatively lower in calories, plus they are easy to season. Your starchy vegetables, like potatoes, rice and corn are a small amount of your plate. These are good for you to eat, but you should eat them in limited amounts – about ½ cup at a meal. Then your plate will have some type of meat product, like chicken or beef. You can eat about 3 ounces at lunch and supper and still be well within your limits. But that is a much smaller portion than you are probably used to eating. This is about eating a balanced meal – the right amounts in relation to each other.

Another thing you can do to help your diet is to eat consistently at the same times every day. Whether you eat 3, 4 or 5 times in a day, you can balance your plate for meals and snacks. If you are used to eating meals and snacks, go ahead and make them fit into the meal plan that you build. But you have to try to make all your meals in a way that helps you improve your health. A sugary snack every now and then will be ok, but those can easily turn into daily things which won't be good for you.

When you have a plan, it's easier to eat the right things and get your meals correct. You have already bought the right things and now you are just working on setting it out for the week. That makes it easy to eat at the same times. Then your body doesn't get too hungry and send you on a "snacking" frenzy. All of this leads to success.

Ok, now that you know how to make a well rounded plate, I want to tell you about the different types of foods and how you should choose what to eat. At the end of the information about how much and how many, I will work through a meal plan example so you can create your own meal pattern.

Reduce Your Protein Intake

We calculated the amount of protein that you should eat in the previous section about protien needs. Now, if you follow my guidance about how to shape your plate in the section about how to eat, you will find it easier to reduce the amount of protein you eat.

Right now, you probably are like most Americans and eat half of your plate with meat or chicken or fish. That is way too much for the average person, and if you have kidney disease, it is really too much. Most of the time you will find yourself with about 2-3 ounces of meat on your plate. That is enough for a person to maintain their health.

For example, if you were to have 60 grams of protein for the day, you could eat it as 10 gm for breakfast, 25 gm for lunch and 25 gm for supper. That would be about 1 egg at breakfast and 3 ounces of meat at each of the other meals. It does not sound like much, but you have plenty of other items on your plate. You will find it easy to fill up because you have lots of vegetables and fruits and a little starch. The raw or frozen fruits and vegetables have lots of fiber in them and keep you feeling full. And if you are not on a fluid restriction, go ahead and drink lots of water. It will also help keep you full.

Manage Your Potassium

Potassium is essential to your health and well-being. It is also an element and an electrolyte that keeps your muscles moving. Your cells need potassium to keep working. So, it seems like you should not have to worry about it, but you really really do. You need to be aware of your potassium levels so you know if you need to reduce the amount you take in or not. Your doctor can tell you this. Just ask you doctor for the amount of potassium that you should take in every day. From that, it will be easy to manage how much.

Use these less often: Higher Potassium Foods	Use these more often: Lower Potassium Foods
Vegetables – Tomatoes, Potatoes, Spinach, Zucchini, Brussels sprouts, Greens, Carrots (raw), Vegetable juices	Vegetables – Olives, cabbage, iceberg lettuce, green beans, onions, Romaine lettuce, beets, green peas
Dried Peas & Beans – black beans, lentil beans, Lima beans, refried beans	White rice, corn tortilla, waffles, rye bread, wild rice
Dried fruits – dates, prunes, raisins	Fruits - Grapes, Mandarin oranges, Plums
Fruits/Juices – Banana, Mango, Oranges, Cantaloupe, Nectarine, Apricots	Fruits – Apples, Blackberries, Cherries, Grapes, Peaches (canned), Pears, Pineapple, Plums, Strawberries, Watermelon, Tangerines
Chocolate (1.5 – 2 ounces)	Hard Candies
Nuts and seeds, peanut butter	Noodles, rice, Bread and bread products that are not whole grain

And if you need to eat less potassium, you will soon find that many vegetables are "off limits" to you because of the amount of potassium they contain. You can learn an easy way to leach your vegetables to get the potassium to a lower level. Leaching vegetables is a way of soaking vegetables to remove some of the potassium they contain.

Some foods that you really want to eat are high potassium foods. It's hard to not eat them because they are a potassium rich foods. You can do several things to lower the amount of potassium and help you in your quest to achieve a low potassium diet. Learning how to leach vegetables to reduce the amount of potassium is a basic skill that is very important to you when cooking for a renal diet. You will need more potassium restriction as your kidney failure worsens, and while on dialysis. So, being able to still eat some of the high potassium foods by leaching vegetables will enable you to continue to have some variety in your diet.

What is leaching? Leaching is the process of removing potassium out of vegetables by soaking and other means so that the vegetable releases some of its potassium instead of ingesting it. Learning how to leach vegetables is a valuable practice for people on a kidney diet to allow for continued variety of foods. Leaching reduces the amount of potassium in vegetables to 25-50% of the original value. The longer you soak them, the warmer the water, and the smaller the pieces makes the difference.

Now, let us get started learning how to leach vegetables.

High potassium foods need to be prepped for eating by leaching the potassium out of them for a period of time. This usually takes about 2-4 hours.

Potatoes, sweet potatoes, carrots, beets and rutabagas require the following process:

1. Prepare a pot with cold water that is large enough to hold the amount of vegetable you are preparing.

2. Peel the vegetable and slice it about 1/8th inch thick (or as thin as you can), place the slices in the cold water to prevent them from turning brown
3. Once you have peeled all the vegetables, empty the pot, and rinse the vegetables in warm water. Then fill the pot back up – using about 10 times the amount of water to the amount of vegetables. If you have 1 cup of potatoes, add 10 cups of water.
4. Cover the pot and let it soak for a minimum of 2 hours. If you soak them for longer, change the water about every 3-4 hours.
5. Once you have allowed them to soak for the time allotted, you should pour out the water and rinse the vegetables again.
6. Cook the vegetable using a ratio of 5:1 for water to vegetables. Again, if you have 1 cup of potatoes, cook them in 5 cups of water.
7. Now you are ready to eat them.

Other high potassium foods that you can process by leaching vegetables are squash, mushrooms, cauliflower and frozen greens. You should do a slightly different process when leaching those vegetables – follow this process:

1. Thaw the frozen vegetables to room temperature and drain the excess water.
2. Rinse the vegetables in warm water. Then fill a pot up – using about 10 times the amount of water to the amount of vegetables.
3. Cover the pot and let it soak for a minimum of 2 hours. If you soak them for longer, change the water about every 3-4 hours.
4. Once you have allowed them to soak for the time allotted, you should pour out the water and rinse the vegetables again.
5. Cook the vegetable using a ratio of 5:1 for water to vegetables. Enjoy them.

I hope that you understand how easy it can be to remove some of the potassium by learning to leach vegetables. This will help you add some variety to your diet without having to eat too many special foods.

Manage Your Phosphorus Intake If Required

Phosphorus is a mineral in our food that our bodies use to create energy and build strong bones. Normally, your kidneys are very good at removing extra amounts of phosphorus from your blood stream and excreting it through your urine. As your kidneys become more damaged, you have a harder time removing phosphorus from your blood stream. This makes your body's natural balance off and results in calcium being removed from your bones to counteract the increased phosphorus levels.

You should start off in the early stages by not drinking dark colored carbonated beverages. These contain a large amount of phosphorus and if they can be avoided, it will help keep your kidneys healthier longer. You most likely won't need to closely watch your phosphorus intake of other foods until you are near stage 4 or 5. At that time, your doctor may also prescribe medications that help your body block the absorption of phosphorus into the blood stream so that you can continue to eat a good variety of foods.

Most foods to avoid are going to be fast foods and those that are highly processed. Reduce your intake of them now to help your kidneys.

Eliminate these : Higher Phosphorus Foods	Use these more often: Lower Phosphorus Foods
Cow's Milk, Pudding, Yogurt- regular and Greek	Rice Milk, Soy Milk, Creamer – ½ and ½
Organ Meats – Oysters, Beef Liver	Poultry, Fish
Beans – Lentils, Black Beans, Soybeans	Vegetables that are low in phos – like wax beans, broccoli, asparagus, carrots, lettuce, onions, green beans, wax beans
Cola (dark colored) drinks	Iced tea made from tea bags, water,

	lemon-lime sodas, gingerale
Soups made with milk	Soups made with broth
Hard Cheeses – cheddar & cottage cheese	Cream cheeses, Brie
Nuts – peanuts, almonds, peanut butter	Popcorn, popsicles, applesauce, fruits – grapes, pears, pineapple, pears
Quick breads (make with baking soda), cornbread, muffins, pancakes, waffles	Bread products that are not whole wheat, and that are refined – bagels, English muffins, croissants
Cereals that are high in fiber – Raisin bran, cheerios, oatmeal	Corn flakes, cream of wheat, Rice chex

Calculating Your Own Meal Plan

{This information can tend to be complicated. I tried to make it as simple as possible. I also provide pre-done meal plans as part of the membership at my website www.renaldiethq.com if you don't want to take the time to do this}

Step 5. Enter the calorie level you determined you needed from step 3 into the blue box on the spread sheet. Choose one of the levels – little or no activity, moderately active, or lose weight. The sheet will calculate out the calorie amounts for you for each of 2 options – just 3 meals, 3 meals and a bedtime snack, or 3 meals and 2 snacks. At this point, you can choose which "meal pattern" will best suit your needs.

Here is where it can get hard to do the right thing and know what that is. I know you understand that a lot of food is going to be limited on this diet. I want you know now that the more work you do now, the better off you are in the future. Every day of limiting your sodium and protein, you are taking a step towards a longer life without dialysis. Let that inspire you to do this well.

I am going to use as an example the male that we calculated the protein and total calories for earlier in the book.

He required 2153 total calories (I will round up to 2200 calories) and 70 grams of protein for the day.

So, I need to think about how he would want to eat. He probably likes 3 meals per day and 2 snacks.

This is how I am going to divide out the day. You will need to figure out how many meals you want per day, divide out the calories by that number and how big you want the meals. The same thing with your protein. Those are the two most important things that we need to consider. We also want to keep our consumption to less than 2000 mg of sodium.

Meal	Calories	Protein
Breakfast	500 calories	10 gm
Lunch	600 calories	25 gm
Midday snack	250 calories	5 gm
Supper	600 calories	25 gm
Evening Snack	250 calories	5 gm

You can see that the totals add up to 2200 calories and 70 gm protein.

Now for the meals. I need to look for items that are good to eat and have low protein, and equal the right amount of calories. You can divide the meals up into different groupings – using general information on food groups.

For example – Diabetic exchanges make a good basic reference point for you to start with. Then you can choose the items in each category based on what is low sodium, low potassium or low phosphorus depending on your needs.

This article by the Mayo clinic explains how diabetic exchanges work and how you can find out serving sizes based on lists. Mayo Clinic Diabetic Exchanges - http://www.renaldiethq.com/idsk

But in addition to breaking out your meal plan by amount of calories and amount of protein, you should balance each meal. You can eat 50% carbohydrate, 20% protein and 30% fat, or you can mix it up another way. I am going to show you using a 50/15/35 (Carb, Protein, Fat). The only problem is that I need to stick to my pre-determined amounts of calories for protein so I am within that limit. So I may need to go higher on carbs or fat.

So, at a meal, I need to break down the total calories into the predetermined ratio. I ended up with a 55/11/34 ratio in my spread sheet.

(Spread sheet with excel calculations is in the file you receive so you can enter your own numbers and get the results)

Meal	Total Calories	Carb Cal	Gm of Carb	% calories from Carb	Protein Cal	Gm of Protein	% calories Pro	Fat Calories	Gm of Fat	% calories Fat
Breakfast	500	260	65	52%	40	10	8%	200	22	40%
Lunch	600	300	75	50%	100	25	17%	200	22	33%
Snack	250	155	39	62%	20	5	8%	75	8	30%
Supper	600	300	75	50%	100	25	17%	200	22	33%
Snack	250	155	39	62%	20	5	8%	75	8	30%
Totals	2200	1170	293	55%	280	70	11%	750	83	34%

Step 6. Using the tab that is called, "Meal Plan", enter the values you want for each meal or snack into the blue fields labeled "Total Calories". Divide the protein that you are allowed for the day throughout the day as well. You can use the amounts that are pre-figured for you from step 5 or divide it up as you see fit. I chose to divide out the day differently than the spreadsheet did. Enter the grams of protein you need per meal in the blue box under Gm of Protein.

Next:

    a. Take the total calories for the meal or snack, and subtract the protein calories for that meal or snack from that number.

    b. Multiply the amount by .6 for the carbohydrate calories. Subtract that amount from the total then you have the calories for fat left.

    c. Enter the amounts into the green boxes under the correct column. The spreadsheet will calculate the rest for you and tell you the grams for each area. (The second spreadsheet on that page automatically calculates the carbohydrate and fat calories for you based on this formula if you want to use that.)

d. Example – I have 500 calories total for the meal, and I have 40 calories for protein. 500-40=460 calories left. I multiply the 460 x 0.60 = 276 calories for carbohydrate. I subtract the carbohydrate calories from the remaining amount: 460-276=184 calories for fat.

    1. If I add up the amounts = 40 + 276 + 184 = 500 calories for the meal.

Now, you have a place to start. The spread sheet that I gave you – all you will have to enter is the total calories by meal, and how many grams of protein you want per meal, and it will calculate for you if you use the 2nd sheet on the page. It also calculates the gm of each category and the % calories from each category. I made the one that doesn't calculate available so you can do it yourself and your own way if you like to go low carb or something.

So, since I am using diabetic exchanges, I know the following: (remember these are generalizations!)

Item	Gm Carb/svg	Gm Protein/svg	Gm Fat/svg	Calories/serving
Starch	15	3	1	80
Fruit	15	0	0	60
Milk (1%)	12	8	1	100
Non-starchy vegetables	5	2	0	25
Meat/Meat Substitutes (medium fat)	0	7	4-7	75
Fat	0	0	5	45

If you go to the Mayo Clinic site, you can find the foods in each category and how they line up. I can't give them all to you here, but you will have that as a resource to use.

Step 7. Figure out how many servings of each category of food you will use per meal using the exchange lists.

For breakfast in my example, I have:

500 calories, 65 gm carbohydrate, 10 gm protein, and 22 gm of fat.

I know that starches have 15 gm of carbohydrate and a little protein. I divide the total amount of carbohydrate allowed by 15 to understand how many servings of carbohydrate I will use at this meal. I have 65 gm of carbohydrate – which is a little over 4 servings. So I will use 45 gm CHO (carbohydrate) – 3 servings of bread will do. I also want 1 serving of fruit, and I will choose ½ cup of mandarin oranges, since they are low potassium.

Did you see what I did? I knew that starches use 15 gm of carbohydrate per serving, and so do juice. I told you before, not to freak out TOO much about vegetable protein. SO the protein in white bread is a little and I will count it but if I am over I am worried about my **animal protein** sources first.

So far I have 3 slices of bread and some mandarin oranges.

I want to know how many servings of protein I can use, so I look at the table again. I have 10 gm for this meal, and 1 ounce of protein has 7 grams of protein. So I have about one ounce of meat or meat substitute to use in this meal. A hard boiled egg sounds good. It's got no carbohydrate and 7 gm of protein. Now I have used up most of my protein for this meal. I have fat as well to use in this meal. Each tsp of butter has 5 gm of fat, so I will use 4 tsp of butter on my 3 pieces of bread. (Better known as 1 Tbsp + 1 tsp). And I will give him water to drink.

Breakfast: 3 slices white bread – 210 cal, 9 gm protein (plant based)
              1 Tbsp + 1 tsp unsalted butter – 200 calories, 0 gm protein
              1 hard boiled egg – 70 calories, 6 gm protein
              ½ cup mandarin oranges, canned – 60 calories, 0 protein
              Beverage – water
              Total: 540 calories, 15 gm protein

Well, my breakfast was a little high on the calories, but I am sure we will make that up in the day.

For lunch in my example, I have:

600 calories, 75 gm carbohydrate, 25 gm protein, and 22 gm of fat.

I have 5 servings of carbohydrate for this meal (I just divided the total number of carbohydrates by 15 to give me the correct number of servings). I have 3.5 ounces of meat servings (7 gm of protein per ounce) and I have 4 servings of fat again. Lunch could be a salad and sandwich meal. The sandwich will be 2 more slices of white bread. Meat for the sandwich would be good as low sodium turkey or low sodium ham. About 3 ounces makes for a good sandwich. I will use mayonnaise on the sandwich, and that counts as a fat. To make it a colorful meal, I will have ½ cup of carrots (5 gm carbs as a non-starchy vegetable), and 1 cup of salad. The salad can be lettuce or romaine , as both are good as low potassium foods. Add more colorful vegetables to the salad – broccoli or cucumbers. Overall it should be about 1.5 cups of salad. That adds about 15 gm more carbohydrate to the menu. Add olive oil and vinegar as the dressing, and using about 1 Tbsp of oil adds 3 more fats to the meal.

Lunch:
2 slices white bread – 140 cal, 4 gm protein
Mayonnaise, 1 Tbsp – 57 calories, 0 gm protein
Turkey Deli Slices (3 ounces) – 60 calories, 21 gm protein
½ cup carrots, cooked – 25 calories, 1 gm protein
1.5 cup salad mixed – 70 calories, 3 gm protein
Olive oil, 1 Tbsp – 150 calories, 0 gm protein
Vinegar or Lemon Juice – 0 calories, 0 gm protein
Apple, 2 medium – 120 calories, 0 gm protein
Total: 622 calories, 29 gm protein

That seems to be a very large lunch, and we are over again on protein – and a tad bit on calories. This is why it is much more of an art and requires a lot of work and thinking.

For the midday snack in my example, I have:

250 calories, 39 gm carbohydrate, 5 gm protein, and 8 gm of fat.

What sounds like a good snack? A piece of fruit and some peanut butter or graham crackers and some nuts? I know that nuts can be high in potassium, but we are also adding just a small amount to our day, so overall we will be able to manage any issues as long as we stay with low potassium foods most of the time. And our main concern is sodium, which we have done a decent job of keeping low for our first two meals.

For this snack, I am going with 2 graham crackers and ½ ounce of dry roasted peanuts. I'm also adding a low potassium fruit to increase calories.

Snack: Graham Crackers, 2 crackers – 70 calories, 1 gm protein
         Peanuts, ½ ounce – 75 calories, 3.5 gm protein
         Peach, 1 small – 60 calories, 1 gm protein
         Total: 205 calories, 4.5 gm protein

Supper meals are usually the larger meal of the day, but for a stage 3-4 kidney disease patient, you may find that lunch is the better meal to have as a large meal. It makes digestion a little easier. And both lunch and supper in this plan are the same amount of calories. So they are easy to interchange.

For supper in my example, I have:

600 calories, 75 gm carbohydrate, 25 gm protein, and 22 gm of fat.

Think about what is a good supper. Earlier in the book, I wrote about making a balanced plate. With ¼ meat, ¼ carbohydrate, and ½ vegetables and fruit. Let's go with that in mind.

How about a 3 ounce (cooked) chicken breast? Sounds good, with some rice. I have the same exchanges of all the food item categories that I had at lunch. I have 5 carbohydrates. So I can use 2 on rice. 2/3 cup of rice – white or wild will make for 30 gm carbohydrate. I can put 2 tsp of butter on the rice. (2 fats) Now, I need to add some vegetables and fruits. I can add 12 spears of asparagus (10 carbohydrate gm), and 1 cup of carrots (10 grams of carbohydrate). That's a lot to eat already. I will just add some grapes to the meal. Every now and then, you add milk or milk products, but limit it to one time per day until you know how your doctor feels about it.

Supper: Chicken breast, 3 ounces – 225 calories, 21 gm protein
         Wild Rice, 2/3 cup – 120 calories, 5 gm protein
         Butter for rice, 2 tsp – 90 calories, 0 g protein
         Asparagus, 12 spears – 50 calories, 1 gm protein
         Carrots, 1 cup – 50 calories, 1 gm protein
         Grapes, 1 cup – 60 calories, 0 gm protein
         Total: 595 calories, 28 gm protein

I also have a snack before bed. For the evening snack in my example, I have:

250 calories, 39 gm carbohydrate, 5 gm protein, and 8 gm of fat.

You might have noticed that I made the lunch and supper meal the same amount and the two snacks the same amount of food. That is not an accident. It makes it easier for you to figure out what to eat and how much when you are working on similar sized meals and portions. But, back to the snack. I had graham crackers and peanuts earlier. I want some breakfast type foods now, so I would eat some cheerios and drink a little juice.

Snack: Cheerios, 1 cup – 110 calories, 3.4 gm protein
                Apple Juice, 1 cup – 120 calories, .5 gm protein
                Total: 230 calories, 3.9 gm protein

You might notice that I am paying close attention to calories and protein, and not necessarily making sure I get all the carbohydrates in there. It's important to you as a renal patient on a restricted diet to know that you are not going over on your protein needs, but also that you get the calories you need so you don't lose weight.

For the day – summary:
Breakfast: 540 calories, 15 gm protein
Lunch: 622 calories, 29 gm protein
Snack: 205 calories, 4.5 gm protein
Supper: 595 calories, 28 gm protein
Snack: 230 calories, 3.9 gm protein
Total: 2192 calories, 80.4 gm protein
Goal: 2200 calories, 70 gm protein

The overage on the protein comes from non-animal sources, so I am not going to get too upset about it. As you can already see, protein is hard to eliminate from your diet. Many foods contain protein in them. You have a plan, and you can arrange your food how you need it for the day using the spreadsheet I gave you in the downloads and the guidelines and information in the other sheets I gave you that contain the information on many types of foods.

Step 8. Plan out how many of each type of food you will have per meal – how many starches, how many vegetables, how many milks, etc. Then assemble your meals using the recommended listing from the Mayo Clinic that shows exchanges – and your spreadsheets showing the low potassium and low sodium foods.

The key to making this work is that you have to read labels and measure/weigh your food so that you know what you are eating. No longer will you be able to just eat the entire container of crackers or soup. You need to get a good understanding of how much you can eat, then, when you are clear on that front you can start to eat without working at it so hard. But, this is a lifestyle change, and you will see results with this method.

Summary of Steps In The Meal Planning Process Using The Spreadsheets

Step 1: Use the provided spreadsheet and enter your numbers to determine your adjusted body weight if needed.

Step 2. At this point, you can **enter your numbers into the spreadsheet** in the blue sections labeled – weight in pounds, height in inches, age in years. Enter your adjusted body weight you just calculated if you are overweight.

Step 3. The spreadsheet automatically gives you the numbers for different activity levels based on your calculated needs. The basic calorie number is the number that you need to lay in bed and rest all day. The little or no activity is a slight increase over your basic calorie needs, and the moderately active number is a greater increase over your baseline number. The lose weight is the little or no activity number with 500 calories per day subtracted.

Step 4. The spreadsheet will calculate this for you automatically. Or you can do it by just taking your (adjusted) weight in pounds, divide by 2.2 to get your weight in kilograms, and multiply by 0.8.

Step 5. Enter the calorie level you determined you needed from step 3 into the blue box on the spreadsheet. Choose one of the levels – little or no activity, moderately active, or lose weight. The sheet will calculate out the calorie amounts for you for each of 2 options – just 3 meals, 3 meals and a bedtime snack, or 3 meals and 2 snacks. At this point, you can choose which "meal pattern" will best suit your needs.

Step 6. Using the tab that is called, "Meal Plan", enter the values you want for each meal or snack into the blue fields labeled "Total Calories". Divide the protein that you are allowed for the day throughout the day as well. You can use the amounts that are pre-figured for you from step 5 or divide it up as you see fit. I chose to divide out the day differently than the spreadsheet did.

Step 7. Figure out how many servings of each category of food you will use per meal using the exchange lists.

Step 8. Plan out how many of each type of food you will have per meal – how many starches, how many vegetables, how many milks, etc. Then assemble your meals using the recommended listing from the Mayo Clinic that shows exchanges – and your spreadsheets showing the low potassium and low sodium foods.

Eating Lower Fat To Reduce Your Risk Of Heart Disease

You should be aware by now that you need to eat lower sodium foods to control your blood pressure. Controlling your blood pressure helps your kidneys. But you also should realize that heart disease goes hand in hand with kidney disease, and it's important to eat a lower amount of saturated fats to help lower your risk.

Saturated fat and trans-fat are both bad for your heart and arteries. Saturated fats are those fats that are solid at room temperature, such as butter and margarine or lard. Trans-fats tend to be solid at room temperature as well, and are used in many baked products to help preserve them longer. Crisco is a good example of trans-fat. You should read labels and avoid ingesting trans-fat if at all possible.

You should eat certain kinds of fat on a kidney diet, it's one of the only ways you can get calories that are not full of protein and potassium. But eat the good fats. When you eat bread, you might want to dip it in olive oil instead of putting butter on it. Use monounsaturated and polyunsaturated fats to cook with – like safflower oil, canola oil and olive oil.

Many things, besides just eating lower saturated fat, will help your heart disease risk. Losing weight, exercising, managing your diabetes are some of the things that will help.

Let's talk about some of the best ways to manage your cardiac and kidney diet.

1. You should learn to do a few things, in terms of eating, that may not be what you are used to. Eating a diet higher in fiber is very helpful with lowering your cholesterol, because fiber can absorb excess cholesterol and helps your digestive system. Because you are a kidney disease patient, you will want to carefully balance eating things like whole wheat bread and white bread. The difference in potassium levels may not be a problem and you can get the extra fiber you need. To get more fiber, you can also eat whole fruits and vegetables – or less processed versions of vegetables and fruits. Such as eating a whole apple instead of applesauce.

2. One of the best sources of fiber is beans, but those can be very hard on a kidney diet. I suggest you look at whether or not you can work them into your diet, because they are very filling and good for your heart. But if you cannot, focus on eating more whole grains, less processed foods in your diet.

3. Eat lower fat food items when given a choice. High fat foods are going to be the fried versions of food, such as fried chicken, fried catfish and French fries. Some lower fat options you have are 1% or skim milk, egg whites or Eggbeaters, vegetables that are steamed with no added butter, skim milk cheese, low fat yogurt, low fat cottage cheese, lean cuts of meat like round and sirloin (limit to 3oz at a time), fish, and poultry without the skin.

4. Use the monounsaturated and polyunsaturated fats more often than saturated fats. Unsaturated fats stay liquid at room temperature. So most of the cooking oils that you see are mainly unsaturated fats – olive oil, canola oil, safflower oil, peanut oil, and sunflower oil. You can also eat mayonnaise, avocados, olives, almonds, and most nuts and seeds. They do have a place in your diet – but you need to be aware of their affect on your kidneys and how much you can eat.

5. Sugar can affect your triglyceride levels, so you should avoid eating high-sugar foods. Simple sugars are easily absorbed into your blood stream, and your liver may use that to make into more triglycerides. Sugar also adds calories to your diet without much nutritional value, so you can end up eating more calories than you realize when you consume things like regular sodas, honey, syrup, fruit drinks, frosting, cake, cookies, candy, pies and pastries. Save them for occasional use, not every day. If you eat something like a fruit – which has mainly fructose – you are better off than drinking juice because you got fiber with the fruit which slows the absorption of the sugar. So that is why whole fruits are much better to eat, even if they contain mainly simple sugars.

6. Limit the amount of alcohol you drink. Alcohol can increase blood triglycerides and has almost as many calories as fat. Talk to your doctor about what amount is healthy for you.

Dining Out For The Kidney Diet

The options when you are eating out are extensive. Many people may prefer to wait until they have a better grasp on the diet before eating out. The challenges related to eating out are the portion sizes and the sodium content of meals, for the most part. Much of the food is high in fat and sugars as well.

But I know it's hard to always eat at home or take your food with you. So, I want to give you some ideas about how to eat out better. And in the files that you downloaded, one of the sets of papers has information on the sodium, protein and calories of foods at common restaurants. Part of it is missing – nothing on potassium or phosphorus, but you can use your knowledge of high potassium foods and apply it here – oranges, potatoes, cantaloupe and bananas, among other things are still high and still should be limited.

Many towns and cities are also requiring nutritional information to be posted so you know how much you are consuming. One of my favorite places to eat is Panera Bread. You can go online to the nutrition calculator: http://www.paneranutrition.com/?ref=/menu/index.php and build the meal you want to eat before you even go to the restaurant.

Which leads me to the next tidbit – planning ahead is your best weapon to stick with your meal plan. Knowing what you are going to eat before you go is invaluable. It allows you to not even be tempted to open the menu – so you don't see all the food you "can't have". If you think of yourself as deprived, that is how you will feel. But why did you go out in the first place? To chat with friends and to see other people? Not to eat so much that it makes you sicker. Food is one of the tools you are using to fight the progression of your kidney disease, and not a punishment or reward.

Eating at restaurants, you can find your best options in the appetizers and salads sections of the menu. Or the kids section if you are lucky. That's because those portion sizes are going to be a bit smaller and you can assemble your meal without having to accept a bunch of side dishes that will not be good for you. The only problem with the appetizers section is that you will have to be careful as most of the foods are fried foods.

In the salads section, you can ask for the dressing to be put on the side, or ask for oil and vinegar to make your own dressing. I personally use lemon juice in combination with a smaller amount of dressing to thin it out and make it cover the majority of the salad. Oil and vinegar don't add sodium, so you will have a lower sodium meal if you choose that. Add a grilled chicken breast to your salad and you are in business!

When you are ordering in a restaurant that you are not familiar with, ask the server questions. I would recommend asking the following:

1. How many ounces is the meat portion?
2. Is there a way to get a "lunch" size portion? (These are usually smaller amounts of the same items)
3. Can you bring me the meal and a box right away – so you can cut it in half and put half of the meal in the box to eat at a later time?
4. Can you substitute the side dishes? (getting rice or noodles instead of potatoes, for example)
5. What are the ingredients in this dish? (to avoid foods that you know you should not have like limiting tomatoes, potatoes, and salt)
6. Can you put the dressings and gravies on the side?

If you want to order a soup and salad, for example, get the broth soup. The cream soup is made with milk or dairy ingredients, and will be higher in potassium. Getting a ½ sandwich is a good way to decrease the amount of meat or animal protein that you eat. Check out the toppings to see if you want to substitute some of them as well, like the tomato and any sort of dressing. Have them served on the side and then add a smaller amount to your food.

Finally, make sure you drink water or unsweetened tea. You should try to keep your beverages so that they are similar to what you drink at home so you don't go overboard on those.

Putting It All Together

Once you have determined your meal plan and worked to get it created just right, I encourage you to consider the following list when trying to balance your meals.

1. Eat fish more often. Most fish is lower in fat and the fat it does have is healthy for you. Flavoring fish is easier too, since much of it is bland (tilapia, cod), so you can add seasonings that make the fish taste great without adding a lot of salt.
2. When choosing the method to cook your meals, choose baking, broiling and roasting for meats instead of frying.
3. Use olive oil or non-stick spray to coat your pans instead of shortening or butter. You should also try to use unsaturated fats in recipes when you can.
4. For flavoring foods, especially vegetables, use lemon juice, vinegar and herbs instead of gravy.
5. Purchase and use low fat cheeses, instead of regular cheeses. Use them in small amounts to add flavor but not smother a dish.
6. Use low-fat yogurt in dishes instead of sour cream when you can – even just substituting half will lower the calories.
7. Instead of choosing high sugar, high fat pastries and pies for desserts – eat fresh fruits. Stop thinking dessert has to be a sweet and you can even skip it sometimes.
8. Trim the excess and visible fat that you see on meats, and pull off the skin from chicken and turkey before you cook them.
9. Eating out is a challenge. Be prepared, know what you are going to eat, and do not let yourself get too hungry so you want to eat everything at the table.

You have some choices to make. Throughout this book, my mission was to teach you how to create your own meal pattern and plan for a stage 3 or 4 kidney disease diet. It's not an easy thing to do, and I tried to make it as easy as possible. The goal of this diet is to lower the protein and sodium that you eat to allow your kidneys to continue to do their job in your body. It's possible to get this diet figured out and keep your kidney disease from progressing further.

I hope that you enjoyed my book, and that you can make your renal diet work for you. You can check out my other related books at Amazon.com on my author page - http://www.amazon.com/Mathea-Ford/e/B008E1E7IS/

Made in the USA
Lexington, KY
04 May 2014